GLP-1 Diet for Women

A Beginner's Guide to Understanding GLP-1 and a 5-Step Plan to Naturally Activate It with Recipes & Meal Plans

mf

copyright © 2025 Isadora Kwon

All rights reserved No part of this book may be reproduced, or stored in a retrieval system, or transmitted in any form or by any means, electronic, mechanical, photocopying, recording, or otherwise, without express written permission of the publisher.

Disclaimer

By reading this disclaimer, you are accepting the terms of the disclaimer in full. If you disagree with this disclaimer, please do not read the guide.

All of the content within this guide is provided for informational and educational purposes only, and should not be accepted as independent medical or other professional advice. The author is not a doctor, physician, nurse, mental health provider, or registered nutritionist/dietician. Therefore, using and reading this guide does not establish any form of a physician-patient relationship.

Always consult with a physician or another qualified health provider with any issues or questions you might have regarding any sort of medical condition. Do not ever disregard any qualified professional medical advice or delay seeking that advice because of anything you have read in this guide. The information in this guide is not intended to be any sort of medical advice and should not be used in lieu of any medical advice by a licensed and qualified medical professional.

The information in this guide has been compiled from a variety of known sources. However, the author cannot attest to or guarantee the accuracy of each source and thus should not be held liable for any errors or omissions.

You acknowledge that the publisher of this guide will not be held liable for any loss or damage of any kind incurred as a result of this guide or the reliance on any information provided within this guide. You acknowledge and agree that you assume all risk and responsibility for any action you undertake in response to the information in this guide.

Using this guide does not guarantee any particular result (e.g., weight loss or a cure). By reading this guide, you acknowledge that there are no guarantees to any specific outcome or results you can expect.

All product names, diet plans, or names used in this guide are for identification purposes only and are the property of their respective owners. The use of these names does not imply endorsement. All other trademarks cited herein are the property of their respective owners.

Where applicable, this guide is not intended to be a substitute for the original work of this diet plan and is, at most, a supplement to the original work for this diet plan and never a direct substitute. This guide is a personal expression of the facts of that diet plan.

Where applicable, persons shown in the cover images are stock photography models and the publisher has obtained the rights to use the images through license agreements with third-party stock image companies.

Table of Contents

Introduction	**8**
How GLP-1 Affects Women's Bodies	**10**
What Is GLP-1 and Why Does It Matter for Women?	10
The Science of Appetite Control, Metabolism, and Fat Storage	11
Why Women May Struggle More with Weight Loss Than Men	13
The Connection Between GLP-1, Estrogen, and Hormones	15
Why Women Gain (and Struggle to Lose) Weight	**18**
The Challenge of Stubborn Fat (Belly, Thighs, & Hips)	18
How Menstrual Cycles, PCOS, and Menopause Affect Weight	19
Emotional Eating & Stress: Why It's Harder for Women	21
GLP-1's Role in Reducing Cravings and Preventing Weight Regain	22
The 5-Step Plan to Naturally Activate GLP-1	**24**
Step 1: Choosing GLP-1-Boosting Foods	24
Step 2: Eating at the Right Times (Meal Timing & Fasting)	30
Step 3: Balancing Macronutrients for Women's Needs	35
Step 4: Exercise to Enhance GLP-1 Activation	39
Step 5: Lifestyle Habits (Stress, Sleep & Gut Health)	42
The GLP-1 Diet for Women – Meal Plans & Recipes	**47**
7-Day Meal Plan for Women of Different Ages & Goals	47
GLP-1-Friendly Breakfast, Lunch, and Dinner Recipes	**51**
Avocado & Veggie Scramble	52
Greek Yogurt Parfait with Berries and Walnuts	53
Overnight Oats with Nut Butter and Banana	54
High-Protein Green Smoothie	55
Sweet Potato & Black Bean Breakfast Bowl	56
Quinoa Kale Salad with Lemon-Tahini Dressing	57

Grilled Chicken Lettuce Wraps	58
Mediterranean Lentil Bowl	59
Salmon & Sweet Potato Bowl	60
Veggie-Packed Tofu Stir-Fry	61
Baked Herb-Crusted Chicken with Veggies	62
Turkey & Spinach Stuffed Peppers	63
Pan-Seared Salmon with Quinoa Pilaf	64
Veggie-Packed Lentil Soup	65
Zucchini Noodles with Turkey Meatballs	66
Snack & Drink Ideas That Support Appetite Control	**67**
Greek Yogurt and Nut Butter Dip with Apple Slices	68
Cucumber Boats with Hummus	69
Roasted Chickpeas	70
Hard-Boiled Egg and Avocado Slices	71
Trail Mix with a Twist	72
Protein-Packed Matcha Latte	73
Fiber-Boosted Green Smoothie	74
Berry Chia Fresca	75
Golden Almond Milk Latte	76
Cucumber Mint Infused Water	77
Tailoring the Plan for Different Life Stages	**78**
GLP-1 and Weight Loss in Your 20s & 30s	78
GLP-1, Hormones, and Metabolism in Your 40s & 50s	80
Managing Weight After Menopause	81
The Emotional Side of Weight Loss & How to Stay Motivated 83	
How Stress and Emotional Eating Affect GLP-1 Levels	83
The Female Mindset Around Weight Loss: How to Make it Sustainable	85
Realistic Expectations and Avoiding Burnout	86
Troubleshooting Common Challenges	**89**
Not Seeing Results? Adjustments for Your Body	89

How to Overcome Hunger, Fatigue, or Energy Dips	91
Signs Your GLP-1 Activation Needs Extra Support	92
Beyond 30 Days – Making the GLP-1 Lifestyle Sustainable	**95**
Transitioning from a Short-Term Plan to a Lifelong Strategy	95
Building Healthy Habits That Last	97
Other Natural Hormone Hacks for Women's Health	98
Conclusion	**101**
FAQs	**104**
References and Helpful Links	**107**

Introduction

Managing body weight is a deeply personal and often challenging experience for many women. Unlike men, women face unique hurdles linked to their biology, hormones, and life stages. From stubborn belly fat to emotional eating driven by stress or hormonal changes, the weight-loss path is rarely straightforward. What works for one person may not work for others, especially when traditional diets take a "one-size-fits-all" approach.

This is where understanding glucagon-like peptide-1, or GLP-1, comes in. GLP-1 is a natural hormone produced in your gut that plays a crucial role in how your body regulates appetite, digestion, and energy storage.

Think of it as your body's internal communicator, signaling your brain when you're full, managing blood sugar, and even encouraging fat to be used as energy. For women, this hormone can be particularly powerful, addressing some of the biological challenges that make weight loss more difficult compared to men.

Hormonal fluctuations, such as those tied to menstrual cycles, pregnancy, menopause, or conditions like polycystic ovary syndrome (PCOS), can often disrupt appetite control and fat storage. By learning how GLP-1 functions and how to activate it naturally, women can harness its potential to control cravings, stabilize energy levels, and make lasting weight management more achievable.

In this guide, we will talk about the following:

- How GLP-1 Affects Women's Bodies
- Why Women Gain (and Struggle to Lose) Weight
- The 5-Step Plan to Naturally Activate GLP-1
- The GLP-1 Diet for Women – Meal Plans & Recipes
- GLP-1-Friendly Breakfast, Lunch, and Dinner Recipes
- Tailoring the Plan for Different Life Stages
- The Emotional Side of Weight Loss & How to Stay Motivated
- Troubleshooting Common Challenges
- Beyond 30 Days – Making the GLP-1 Lifestyle Sustainable

By the end of this guide, you'll not only understand how GLP-1 impacts your body but also feel empowered to make smarter choices that support your health and well-being for the long term.

How GLP-1 Affects Women's Bodies

Understanding how the body regulates hunger, metabolism, and weight is key to creating strategies that work. For women, these processes can be uniquely complex due to the influence of hormones like estrogen and the role of GLP-1 (glucagon-like peptide-1).

This chapter explores how GLP-1 impacts women's health, its connection to appetite control, and why hormonal differences shape the weight-loss challenges many women face.

What Is GLP-1 and Why Does It Matter for Women?

GLP-1 is a hormone produced in the gut that plays a pivotal role in regulating blood sugar, curbing appetite, and promoting feelings of fullness after eating. It's part of the body's natural system for maintaining energy balance, signaling the brain when to eat and when to stop.

GLP-1's Core Functions

- *Appetite Regulation*: GLP-1 slows the emptying of food from your stomach, making you feel full longer. It also interacts with the brain's hunger centers to reduce cravings.
- *Blood Sugar Control*: After eating, GLP-1 helps release insulin (the hormone that lowers blood sugar) and suppresses glucagon (which raises it), keeping levels stable.
- *Metabolism Support*: By enhancing insulin sensitivity and moderating food intake, GLP-1 contributes to overall energy balance and weight management.

Why Women Benefit from GLP-1 Awareness

Women's fluctuating hormones throughout the menstrual cycle, pregnancy, and menopause can affect GLP-1 production and how effectively it regulates hunger. Knowing this connection empowers women to work with their bodies instead of battling against biological processes. For example, lifestyle strategies that promote healthy GLP-1 activity, such as eating balanced meals and engaging in exercise, can be particularly beneficial.

The Science of Appetite Control, Metabolism, and Fat Storage

Achieving and maintaining a healthy weight isn't just about willpower or discipline. Women face distinct biological mechanisms that influence how they eat, store fat, and burn calories.

Appetite Control Basics

Hunger is regulated by a complex interplay of hormones in the gut and brain. GLP-1 is just one of several hormones involved, working alongside ghrelin (the hunger hormone) and leptin (the satiety hormone). Together, these signals tell your brain whether your body needs fuel or has had enough to eat.

- *GLP-1's Appetite-Suppressing Role*: By slowing digestion and sending satiety signals to the brain, GLP-1 reduces the urge to overeat.
- *Challenges for Women*: Hormonal shifts, especially related to estrogen levels, can affect how hunger and fullness hormones function. During certain phases of the menstrual cycle or in times of stress, women may feel an elevated desire to eat even when their energy needs haven't increased.

Metabolism Myths vs. Reality

Metabolism refers to the chemical processes that convert food into energy. Women often have a slower resting metabolic rate than men, meaning their bodies burn fewer calories at rest. Here's why:

- *Lower Muscle Mass*: Women naturally have less muscle than men, and muscle burns more calories than fat.
- *Hormonal Influence*: Hormones like estrogen and progesterone can slow metabolism during specific life stages, such as menopause.

Fat Storage and Distribution

Women's bodies are biologically programmed to store fat more efficiently than men's, primarily for reproductive purposes. This storage often occurs in areas like the hips, thighs, and lower abdomen, where it's harder to shed. Though this evolutionary process supports fertility and pregnancy, it can make weight loss feel disproportionately challenging compared to men.

Why Women May Struggle More with Weight Loss Than Men

It can be frustrating to feel like weight-loss efforts yield slower results compared to men. Science offers an explanation rooted in biology and hormones.

1. **Gender Differences in Energy Expenditure**

    Men typically burn more calories than women, largely due to differences in muscle mass, body composition, and overall body size. Muscle tissue requires more energy to maintain than fat, so individuals with higher muscle mass naturally have a higher resting metabolic rate.

Even during exercise, men tend to burn calories more efficiently because their bodies are designed to use energy differently, giving them a metabolic advantage. Hormonal differences, such as higher testosterone levels in men, also contribute to increased muscle development and calorie expenditure compared to women.

2. **Hormonal Variability**

Women's hormone levels fluctuate throughout their lives, from monthly menstrual cycles to the hormonal shifts of pregnancy and menopause. These fluctuations can affect appetite, fat storage, and metabolism.

- *Menstrual Cycle*: Elevated progesterone during the luteal phase can increase hunger and cravings, particularly for calorie-rich foods.
- *Menopause*: Declining estrogen levels can result in increased belly fat and a slower metabolic rate.

3. **The Psychological Toll of Societal Expectations**

Cultural pressures around weight loss often place an immense burden on women, making the process even more challenging. Society frequently promotes unrealistic beauty standards, glorifying unattainable ideals that can leave women feeling inadequate or judged. This pressure can lead to extreme measures, such as restrictive diets, which not only intensify emotional stress but can also disrupt hormonal balance and overall health.

Over time, these restrictive behaviors may trigger a frustrating cycle of dieting, temporary weight loss, and rebound weight gain, leaving women both physically and emotionally drained. Addressing these societal expectations is critical to fostering a healthier, more supportive environment for women on their wellness journeys.

The Connection Between GLP-1, Estrogen, and Hormones

GLP-1 doesn't work in isolation; it interacts with other hormones, particularly estrogen, which plays a pivotal role in women's health and metabolism. Understanding these connections provides insights into why women face unique weight-loss challenges.

1. **Estrogen's Role in Fat Storage**

   During childbearing years, estrogen helps direct fat storage to the hips and thighs for reproductive purposes. However, as estrogen levels decline during menopause, fat distribution often shifts to the abdominal area. This change makes weight maintenance more difficult and increases health risks.

2. **Estrogen and GLP-1 Sensitivity**

   Research suggests that estrogen enhances GLP-1's appetite-suppressing effects. This explains why some women experience increased hunger and reduced satiety during menopause, as estrogen levels drop. Supporting GLP-1 activity through diet and exercise becomes even more important during this phase of life.

3. **Hormonal Stress Responses**

   Chronic stress elevates cortisol, a hormone that not only promotes fat storage but also interferes with GLP-1's ability to regulate appetite and blood sugar effectively. This creates a double challenge for women under prolonged stress.

   Women's weight-loss journeys are shaped by unique biological, hormonal, and metabolic factors that require tailored strategies. Far from being barriers, these differences offer an opportunity to approach health and weight management with more knowledge and care.

By understanding the role of GLP-1 in appetite regulation, the effects of estrogen on fat storage, and the natural metabolic challenges women face, you can create a plan that works with your body—not against it. Every woman's body is different, and success comes from developing a sustainable approach that honors your individual needs. With the right tools and mindset, achieving your health goals becomes not just possible but empowering.

Why Women Gain (and Struggle to Lose) Weight

Many women face challenges when trying to lose weight, but the problem runs much deeper than "eating less and exercising more." Weight gain and fat retention in women are influenced by hormones, biological differences, and emotional factors, making it harder to lose weight compared to men. By breaking down the science and offering insights, we can better understand these challenges.

The Challenge of Stubborn Fat (Belly, Thighs, & Hips)

Women often notice that fat accumulates in specific areas, especially:

- Belly
- Thighs
- Hips

This isn't random; it's biology. Women's bodies are designed to store fat in these regions as energy reserves for pregnancy and breastfeeding. The fat in areas like the thighs and hips is mostly subcutaneous fat, which is harder to burn compared to visceral fat (the kind found in the belly).

Belly fat, however, becomes more common as women age, particularly after menopause. When estrogen levels drop, fat tends to shift toward the abdomen. This shift not only affects appearance but also increases health risks, as abdominal fat is known to raise the likelihood of heart disease and diabetes.

Fat retention in these areas is tough to address with standard dieting. It often requires a strategy tailored to work with women's unique biology rather than against it.

How Menstrual Cycles, PCOS, and Menopause Affect Weight

Hormonal fluctuations play a major role in how women gain and lose weight. These shifts occur naturally during menstrual cycles and more significantly with conditions like PCOS or life stages such as **menopause**.

Menstrual Cycle

During the menstrual cycle, hormones like **estrogen** and **progesterone** fluctuate. This impacts weight in several ways:

- *Water retention*: Many women notice extra bloating and temporary weight gain.

- *Cravings*: Hormonal dips can lead to heightened cravings for sugary or high-carb foods, especially before and during menstruation.

While these changes are cyclical, they can create challenges for maintaining consistent weight loss.

PCOS (Polycystic Ovary Syndrome)

PCOS is a common hormonal disorder that affects many women, and it makes weight loss harder for several reasons:

- *Insulin resistance*: This makes the body store fat more easily.
- *Hormonal imbalances*: These can boost appetite or lead to fat storage in the abdominal area.
- *Slower metabolism*: Many women with PCOS need to work harder than average to lose the same amount of weight.

Menopause

Menopause is a game-changer for weight management. Key issues include:

- *Lower estrogen levels*: These cause fat to shift from the hips and thighs to the belly.
- *Slower metabolism*: Aging naturally reduces your metabolic rate, so your body burns fewer calories overall.

- *Loss of muscle mass*: This further reduces metabolism and increases the percentage of body fat.

Understanding that these hormonal shifts are biological—not personal failures—is key to finding effective solutions.

Emotional Eating & Stress: Why It's Harder for Women

Beyond biology, women often face emotional and psychological barriers to weight loss. Stress, in particular, can fuel weight gain through emotional eating and hormonal changes.

Stress and Weight Gain

When you're feeling stressed, your body produces cortisol, often referred to as the "stress hormone." This hormone increases your appetite and can lead to cravings for comfort foods, typically those high in sugar and fat. Chronic stress also encourages fat storage, especially around the belly.

Emotional Eating

Women are more likely than men to turn to food for emotional comfort. This relationship with food can lead to cycles of overeating and self-blame, making weight loss feel like an uphill battle.

Being aware of these patterns and finding alternative coping mechanisms, such as exercise, mindfulness, or therapy, can help break the cycle.

GLP-1's Role in Reducing Cravings and Preventing Weight Regain

While there are significant challenges for women when it comes to weight loss, GLP-1 offers hope. This powerful hormone can help level the playing field by addressing some of the core issues women face.

How GLP-1 Helps

- ***Reduces cravings***: GLP-1 can suppress appetite by sending signals to the brain that you're full. This can help reduce binge eating and make it easier to stick to a healthy eating plan.
- ***Regulates blood sugar***: By balancing blood sugar levels, GLP-1 lowers the chance of energy crashes that often lead to overeating.
- ***Slows stomach emptying***: This keeps you feeling full longer and helps prevent overeating.
- ***Supports long-term weight management***: By curbing hunger and regulating metabolism, GLP-1-based interventions can also reduce the risk of weight regain after initial weight loss.

For women dealing with hormonal challenges, GLP-1 therapies or strategies that boost GLP-1 production (such as high-fiber foods and meal timing) can be game-changers.

Weight management for women isn't about trying harder; it's about working smarter. Understanding how your body works and incorporating strategies that align with your hormones, needs, and emotions can make all the difference.

The 5-Step Plan to Naturally Activate GLP-1

If you're looking for ways to support weight loss, control cravings, and improve overall health, activating GLP-1 naturally is a great place to start. GLP-1 (glucagon-like peptide-1) is a hormone that controls appetite and helps regulate blood sugar. The best part? You can stimulate it naturally through smart choices in food, activity, and lifestyle. Let's break it down into five actionable steps.

Step 1: Choosing GLP-1-Boosting Foods

The foods you choose to eat play a huge role in how your body produces and utilizes GLP-1, a hormone crucial for appetite control and blood sugar regulation. By adding certain nutrient-dense foods to your diet, you can naturally encourage GLP-1 production. This isn't about following a strict meal plan; it's about understanding what fuels your body best and making small, intentional adjustments to your diet.

1. **High-Fiber Foods**

   Fiber is a superstar when it comes to promoting GLP-1. High-fiber foods slow digestion, which gives your gut more time to release GLP-1 into your bloodstream. They also help keep you feeling full for longer, reducing the likelihood of overeating or snacking on less-healthy options.

   Some fantastic high-fiber options include:

   - *Whole grains*: Quinoa, brown rice, oats, and farro.
   - *Vegetables*: Broccoli, cauliflower, leafy greens, carrots, and Brussels sprouts.
   - *Fruits*: Apples, pears, raspberries, and blueberries are all rich in fiber and naturally sweet.
   - *Legumes*: Lentils, chickpeas, black beans, and kidney beans are excellent sources of both fiber and plant-based protein.

   How it helps: Fiber-rich foods feed the beneficial bacteria in your gut, supporting a healthy microbiome. A thriving gut microbiome boosts GLP-1 production, making these foods an excellent foundation for hormonal balance.

   Ideas to try:

- Start your day with a bowl of overnight oats topped with fresh berries and a sprinkle of chia seeds.
- For lunch, try a quinoa salad mixed with roasted vegetables, chickpeas, and a drizzle of olive oil.
- Snack on sliced apple wedges paired with almond butter.

2. **Healthy Fats**

Healthy fats do more than add flavor to your meals; they promote stable blood sugar levels, which helps your body optimize GLP-1 production. They're also essential for absorbing fat-soluble vitamins (like A, D, E, and K) that support overall hormonal health.

Some great sources of healthy fats include:

- *Avocado*: Versatile and packed with heart-healthy monounsaturated fats.
- *Nuts*: Almonds, walnuts, and cashews are nutrient-dense and easy to snack on.
- *Seeds*: Flaxseeds, chia seeds, and sunflower seeds are great for adding texture to meals.
- *Olive oil*: Rich in antioxidants and perfect for dressings, dips, and light sautéing.
- *Fatty fish*: Salmon, mackerel, and sardines are loaded with omega-3 fatty acids, which support endocrine and metabolic health.

How it helps: Healthy fats enhance GLP-1's activity by keeping blood sugar levels steady. Additionally, they slow the absorption of glucose into your bloodstream, improving insulin sensitivity.

Ideas to try:

- Mash an avocado onto a slice of whole-grain toast, sprinkle with pumpkin seeds, and top with a soft-boiled egg for a balanced breakfast or snack.
- Toss a handful of walnuts or almonds into your Greek yogurt with fresh fruit.
- Dress roasted Brussels sprouts or kale with a mix of olive oil, lemon juice, and garlic.

3. **Lean Proteins**

Protein is a powerful macronutrient that stimulates GLP-1 secretion. Eating enough protein not only supports muscle repair but also keeps you feeling full and satisfied for longer periods.

Excellent sources of lean protein include:

- *Eggs*: Packed with nutrients and easy to incorporate into any meal.
- *Poultry*: Skinless chicken and turkey are low in fat and high in protein.
- *Fish*: Salmon, cod, and tilapia are excellent choices that are also rich in omega-3s.

- ***Plant-based proteins***: Lentils, chickpeas, tofu, and tempeh are great options for vegetarians or anyone hoping to diversify their protein sources.

How it helps: Protein slows the release of sugar into the bloodstream, reducing spikes and crashes that interfere with GLP-1 activity. It also partners with fiber to create a slow-digesting, satisfying meal that keeps hunger at bay.

Ideas to try:

- Start your day with a veggie scramble made with eggs, spinach, and mushrooms.
- Grill some chicken or salmon and pair it with a side of roasted sweet potatoes and asparagus for dinner.
- For a snack, enjoy a small bowl of hummus with raw vegetable sticks like celery, carrots, and bell peppers.

4. **Fermented Foods**

Fermented foods are not just trendy; they're a fantastic way to support your gut health, which ties directly into GLP-1 production. These foods contain probiotics, beneficial bacteria that keep your digestive system running smoothly and may even enhance the release of GLP-1.

Top fermented options include:

- *Yogurt*: Choose plain Greek yogurt for a protein-packed snack that also supports gut health.
- *Kefir*: A tangy, drinkable yogurt rich in probiotics.
- *Kimchi*: A spicy, fermented cabbage dish popular in Korean cuisine.
- *Sauerkraut*: Fermented cabbage that's loaded with good bacteria.
- *Miso*: A fermented soybean paste used in soups, marinades, or dressings.

How it helps: A healthy gut microbiome increases GLP-1 secretion and improves insulin sensitivity. It also combats inflammation, which can support other weight management and overall health goals.

Ideas to try:

- Add a dollop of plain yogurt to your breakfast bowl or blend it into a smoothie with spinach and frozen berries.
- Mix kimchi or sauerkraut into your lunchtime salad or use it as a topping for roasted vegetables.
- Make a miso dressing for your favorite salad or drizzle it over grilled fish.

Foods to Avoid

While adding GLP-1-boosting foods to your diet, it's equally important to avoid foods that work against your goals. Refined sugars, processed snacks, and simple carbohydrates can lead to blood sugar spikes and crashes, making it harder for your body to produce GLP-1 effectively. Think white bread, soda, packaged cookies, and sugary cereals. Instead, focus on whole, minimally processed alternatives.

You don't need to overhaul your pantry overnight. Begin with one small change, like replacing your afternoon snack of chips or cookies with a high-fiber fruit and a handful of almonds. Over time, you'll find these adjustments becoming habits that naturally enhance your GLP-1 levels, leading to better appetite control and a more balanced approach to eating.

By filling your plate with whole, nutrient-dense foods, you're setting the foundation for success—not just for activating GLP-1, but for improving your overall health and well-being.

Step 2: Eating at the Right Times (Meal Timing & Fasting)

When it comes to boosting your GLP-1 levels naturally, when you eat is just as important as what you eat. By being thoughtful about your meal timing and incorporating fasting periods, you can help your body optimize GLP-1 production, manage hunger, and stabilize blood sugar levels. These strategies work with your body's natural rhythms, making it easier to control cravings and improve overall health.

How Meal Timing and Fasting Impact GLP-1

GLP-1 is released in your gut in response to food, but your production levels can vary depending on how often you eat and the duration of breaks between meals.

- *Frequent snacking*: Eating every hour or so may not give your body enough time to process food and release GLP-1 efficiently.
- *Meal spacing and fasting*: Allowing longer breaks between meals encourages your body to produce GLP-1, which signals fullness and helps regulate blood sugar.

By eating at set times and including fasting periods, you're giving your digestive system time to work efficiently, which supports more consistent GLP-1 release.

Practical Strategies for Meal Timing

Here's how you can tweak your meal timing to naturally activate GLP-1 and support your weight loss and overall health goals:

1. *Eat with Purpose*: Instead of grazing throughout the day, stick to structured meals. This helps your body anticipate and regulate hormone production.

- Aim for 2-3 main meals each day with 3-4 hours between each meal.
- Avoid mindless snacking between meals; if you need something, choose a small, high-protein option.

<u>Example Meal Schedule:</u>

- *7 a.m.*: Breakfast (oatmeal with berries and almond butter)
- *12 p.m.*: Lunch (grilled chicken, quinoa, and roasted vegetables)
- *6 p.m.*: Dinner (salmon, sweet potatoes, and sautéed spinach)

2. *Front-Load Your Eating*: Your body processes food more efficiently earlier in the day. By consuming most of your calories during breakfast and lunch, you give your metabolism a boost. This strategy is often referred to as **"eating with your circadian rhythm."**
   - Make breakfast and lunch your largest meals.
   - Keep dinner lighter, focusing on protein and vegetables.
3. *Stop Eating Late at Night*: Your digestive system slows down as the day progresses, which can interfere with GLP-1 production if you eat too close to bedtime. Aim to finish your final meal at least 3 hours before going to sleep.

Incorporating Intermittent Fasting

Intermittent fasting (IF) is a popular approach to meal timing that can enhance GLP-1 activation. The goal is to alternate between periods of eating and fasting, giving your body time to reset and balance hormones.

Common Intermittent Fasting Schedules

1. *12/12 Method*: This beginner-friendly approach involves fasting for 12 hours overnight and eating during the other 12 hours.
   - Example schedule: Stop eating at 7 p.m. and have your first meal at 7 a.m.
2. *16/8 Method*: This method extends your fasting window to 16 hours, with an 8-hour eating window. Many find this effective for balancing blood sugar and appetite.
   - Example schedule: Stop eating at 7 p.m. and have your first meal at 11 a.m.
3. *5:2 Method:* For five days of the week, you eat as you normally would. On the other two days, you reduce calorie intake significantly (e.g., 500-600 calories).

Both structured meal timing and fasting encourage GLP-1 activation by creating natural periods where your body isn't digesting food. This allows the hormone to work without interruption.

Tips for Getting Started

If you're new to changing your meal timing, ease into it with these simple steps.

- ***Start with the 12/12 fasting method.*** It's easy to incorporate into your routine since you're asleep during much of the fasting window.
- ***Gradually increase fasting periods.*** If you want to try a longer fasting window, like 16/8, build up to it slowly by extending your overnight fast by an hour every few days.
- ***Don't skip breakfast if it disrupts your routine.*** While fasting can be effective, it's more important to prioritize flexibility and sustainability in your habits.

Supporting Your Eating Window

During your eating window, focus on nutrient-dense meals that include high-fiber foods, lean proteins, and healthy fats. Pairing meal timing with the right food choices maximizes GLP-1 production and keeps you satisfied throughout the day.

Sample Eating Schedule for Beginners (12/12 Method):

- ***7 a.m.***: Breakfast (Greek yogurt with granola and fresh fruit)
- ***12 p.m.***: Lunch (quinoa bowl with black beans, avocado, and sautéed veggies)
- ***7 p.m.***: Dinner (grilled chicken with roasted Brussels sprouts and mashed cauliflower)

Find an eating schedule that fits your lifestyle while giving your body regular breaks between meals. Simple changes, like avoiding late-night snacks or spacing meals evenly, can activate your GLP-1 and support your health. Start small, stay consistent, and take control of your well-being!

Step 3: Balancing Macronutrients for Women's Needs

The way you balance protein, carbs, and fats in your meals has a big impact on your energy levels, how full you feel, and how your hormones, like GLP-1, work. For women, finding the right combination of these nutrients is especially important because it helps keep your hunger in check and supports overall hormone balance.

Here's how to make macronutrients work for you:

Protein First

Protein is your best friend when it comes to GLP-1 production. It not only helps activate GLP-1, but it also keeps you feeling full and prevents cravings later in the day. Women often need around 20-30 grams of protein per meal to get these benefits.

Examples of protein-packed foods:

- Grilled chicken or turkey
- Eggs or egg whites

- Greek yogurt or cottage cheese
- Plant-based options like lentils, chickpeas, or tofu

By making protein the centerpiece of your meal, you're giving your body the support it needs to regulate hunger hormones and stay satisfied longer.

Tip: Start your day with scrambled eggs and spinach or enjoy a quinoa salad with grilled salmon for lunch. Both are simple and protein-packed options!

Choose Healthy Carbs

Carbs are essential for energy, but it's important to focus on the right kind. Complex carbohydrates, which are high in fiber, provide a steady energy source and help stabilize blood sugar levels. This balance supports GLP-1 production, making it easier for your body to manage hunger.

Best options for healthy carbs:

- Whole grains like oats, quinoa, or barley
- Starchy vegetables like sweet potatoes or butternut squash
- Fruits such as apples, berries, or oranges

On the other hand, refined carbs like white bread, pastries, and sugary snacks can cause quick blood sugar spikes followed by crashes, making it harder to keep your hormones balanced.

Tip: Pair your favorite protein with a fiber-rich carb, like roasted sweet potatoes and sautéed greens, for a meal that feeds your body and balances your hormones.

Don't Skip the Fats

Healthy fats are a key part of any balanced meal. They keep you full, help your body absorb essential vitamins, and promote blood sugar stability, which supports GLP-1 activation. However, because fats are high in calories, it's important to watch portion sizes.

Great sources of healthy fats include:

- Avocado slices
- A drizzle of olive oil on your salad or veggies
- A handful of almonds, walnuts, or seeds
- Fatty fish like salmon or mackerel

Tip: Add half an avocado to your lunch salad or dress roasted vegetables with olive oil and lemon juice for a satisfying and nutrient-rich boost.

Keep Hormones in Balance

For women, balancing macronutrients isn't just about satisfying hunger or fueling workouts. It's also essential for keeping hormones in check. Eating too many refined carbs or unhealthy fats can disrupt your body's natural processes, making it harder to activate GLP-1. Instead, aim for meals that include a mix of all three macronutrients to support steady energy and hormone balance throughout the day.

Example of a balanced meal:

- Grilled chicken breast (protein)
- Quinoa (healthy carb)
- Steamed broccoli drizzled with olive oil (fiber + fat)

A Simple Strategy

A great way to balance macronutrients is by following the "plate method." Visualize your plate divided into sections:

- Half the plate is filled with vegetables or leafy greens.
- One quarter is lean protein like chicken, fish, tofu, or eggs.
- The final quarter is a fiber-packed carb like quinoa, brown rice, or sweet potatoes.
- Add a small amount of healthy fat, like avocado or nuts, for extra flavor and fullness.

Balancing your meals this way helps your body activate GLP-1 while giving you the energy and nutrients you need to feel your best. Start small by rethinking one meal a day, and over time, you'll notice how this approach makes a difference in how you feel!

Step 4: Exercise to Enhance GLP-1 Activation

Exercise isn't just good for building strength or burning calories. It also plays a key role in how your body produces and uses hormones like GLP-1, which helps control appetite and regulate blood sugar. By being active, you're giving your body a natural boost that supports weight management and overall health. You don't need an intense or time-consuming workout routine to see the benefits.

How Exercise Impacts GLP-1

When you're physically active, your muscles and cells work more efficiently, which can stimulate the release of GLP-1. Even light movement supports better digestion and hormone balance. The trick is to choose exercises that feel good for your body and fit into your daily routine.

Types of Exercise for GLP-1 Activation

1. *High-Intensity Interval Training (HIIT)*: HIIT exercises feature brief, high-intensity activity interspersed with short recovery intervals. This approach has been shown to boost GLP-1 levels and provides an effective way to raise your heart rate and burn calories efficiently.

   Examples of HIIT exercises:

   - Sprint for 30 seconds, then walk for 90 seconds. Repeat 6-8 times.

- Do 20 seconds of bodyweight exercises like jumping jacks, burpees, or mountain climbers, followed by 40 seconds of rest.

How to start: If you're new to HIIT, try it for just 10-15 minutes a few times a week. Customize the intensity and duration to match your fitness level.

2. ***Strength Training***: Strength training doesn't just build muscle; it also prompts your body to use energy more effectively and boosts metabolism. By lifting weights or doing resistance exercises, you can help your body produce and utilize GLP-1 more efficiently.

   Examples of strength training exercises:
   - Bodyweight exercises like squats, push-ups, or planks.
   - Dumbbell exercises like bicep curls, deadlifts, or tricep extensions.
   - Resistance band exercises for arms, legs, or core.

   How to start: Begin with 2-3 sessions per week. Focus on major muscle groups and aim for 8-12 repetitions of each exercise. If lifting weights feels intimidating, resistance bands are a beginner-friendly option.

3. ***Daily Movement***: Building physical activity into your daily routine can have a surprisingly big impact on your health and GLP-1 activation. You don't need a gym for this one—even light movement can make a difference.

   Simple ways to move daily:

   - Take a 10-15 minute walk after meals to support digestion and encourage steady GLP-1 release.
   - Stretch or do yoga in the morning or after work to improve flexibility and reduce stress.
   - Use the stairs instead of the elevator or add active breaks during your workday.

   How to start: Make small changes like parking farther away, taking short active breaks throughout the day, or setting a daily goal for steps.

   Tips for Building an Exercise Routine

   - ***Start small***: If you're new to exercise, begin with just 10 minutes a day. Even brief efforts add up over time.
   - ***Mix it up***: Combine cardio (like HIIT or walking), strength training, and gentle movements (like yoga or stretching) for a balanced routine.
   - ***Be consistent***: Regular, moderate movement is more effective than occasional intense

workouts. Aim for activities you enjoy and can stick with long-term.

- ***Listen to your body***: Rest when you need to, and gradually increase intensity as your fitness improves.

You don't need to overhaul your routine overnight. Start with something simple, like a short, 10-minute walk after dinner. This small, consistent habit can make a noticeable difference over time. Once you're ready, add in other forms of exercise at your own pace.

By staying active and experimenting with different types of movement, you're supporting your body's natural ability to produce GLP-1. Not only will you feel stronger and more energized, but you'll also be taking an important step toward better health. All it takes is a little action every day!

Step 5: Lifestyle Habits (Stress, Sleep & Gut Health)

Your daily habits have a powerful influence on how your body produces and uses GLP-1. If you're constantly stressed, lacking sleep, or ignoring your gut health, it can disrupt hormone regulation, including GLP-1. But by taking small, manageable steps to care for yourself, you can naturally support this hormone and improve your overall well-being.

1. **Managing Stress**

   Stress is a part of life, but when it's constant, it can increase cortisol levels, interfering with hormones like GLP-1. Chronic stress not only makes you feel overwhelmed but can also lead to overeating and blood sugar imbalances. Finding ways to relax can help get your hormones back on track.

   Simple stress-reducing techniques:

   - *Deep breathing exercises*: Take 5 deep breaths, inhaling through your nose for 4 seconds, holding for 4 seconds, and exhaling through your mouth for 4 seconds. It's a quick way to calm your mind.
   - *Meditation*: Even just 5 minutes of quiet meditation or mindfulness each day can help lower stress levels. Apps like Calm or Headspace can guide you if you're a beginner.
   - *Yoga or gentle stretching*: These activities help release built-up tension in your body while promoting relaxation.

   How to start:

   Add a quick 10-minute stress-relief activity to your daily routine, whether it's a walk outside, deep breathing, or a short yoga session. Over time, this small habit can have a big impact.

2. Prioritizing Sleep

Sleep isn't just about feeling rested. It's also crucial for hormone regulation. When you don't get enough quality sleep, it can throw off your hunger hormones, including GLP-1, and make cravings harder to resist. Aim to prioritize both the quantity and quality of your rest.

Tips for better sleep:

- *Stick to a schedule*: Go to bed and wake up at the same time every day, even on weekends.
- *Establish a soothing bedtime routine* by engaging in calming activities such as reading, gentle stretching, or enjoying peaceful music.
- *Limit screen time*: Avoid screens 1 hour before bed, as the blue light can interfere with melatonin, the hormone that helps you sleep.
- *Make your bedroom sleep-friendly*: Keep it cool, dark, and quiet. Blackout curtains or a white noise machine can help.
- *How to start*: Start small by setting a consistent bedtime each night. If screens before bed are a challenge, try switching to an activity like journaling or reading for 15 minutes before sleep instead.

3. **Supporting Gut Health**

   Your gut plays a major role in GLP-1 production. A healthy microbiome, which is made up of the good bacteria in your gut, can enhance hormone regulation. On the other hand, an unhealthy gut can hinder GLP-1 activation and impact your digestion.

   <u>**Ways to improve gut health:**</u>

   - *Eat probiotic-rich foods*: Include foods like yogurt, kefir, sauerkraut, kimchi, or miso in your diet to add beneficial bacteria to your gut.
   - *Focus on fiber*: High-fiber foods, such as whole grains, vegetables, fruits, and legumes, help keep your gut bacteria fed and thriving.
   - *Stay hydrated*: Drinking plenty of water supports digestion and gut health. Aim for 6-8 cups of water a day.
   - *How to start*: Add one gut-friendly food to your meals each day. For example, enjoy Greek yogurt with breakfast or add some sauerkraut to your salad or sandwich at lunch.

Combine Small Changes for Big Results

Healthy habits don't have to feel overwhelming. You don't need to tackle stress, sleep, and gut health all at once. Start with just one small change, like setting a consistent bedtime or adding a relaxing activity to your routine, and build from there.

An easy place to begin:

- ***Stress relief***: Take a short walk or try a breathing exercise during your lunch break.
- ***Sleep improvement***: Swap evening screen time for a calming cup of herbal tea and a book.
- ***Gut health***: Add a handful of fiber-rich nuts or a piece of fruit to your afternoon snack.

Remember, consistency is more important than perfection. Healthy habits take time, and progress can be slow at first, but even small steps can bring big benefits over time. By managing stress, prioritizing restful sleep, and supporting your gut health, you're helping your body activate GLP-1 naturally and set the foundation for long-term health.

The GLP-1 Diet for Women – Meal Plans & Recipes

In this chapter, we will discuss meal plans and recipes that can help boost GLP-1 levels and support overall gut health in women. These meal plans and recipes are designed to be simple, delicious, and easy to incorporate into your daily routine.

7-Day Meal Plan for Women of Different Ages & Goals

To get started, here is a 7-day meal plan for women of different ages and goals. This meal plan includes breakfast, lunch, snacks, and dinner options that incorporate gut-friendly foods and help activate GLP-1 naturally.

Day 1

Breakfast: Overnight oats with Greek yogurt, chia seeds, berries, and honey

Lunch: Quinoa salad with roasted vegetables and avocado

Snack: Sliced apples paired with almond butter

Dinner: Salmon grilled to perfection, served alongside steamed broccoli and a portion of brown rice

Day 2

Breakfast: Whole grain toast with mashed avocado, finished with a poached egg on top

Lunch: A hearty bowl of lentil soup served alongside whole grain crackers

Snack: Carrot sticks with hummus

Dinner: Baked chicken with roasted sweet potatoes and green beans

Day 3

Breakfast: Greek yogurt parfait with granola and mixed berries

Lunch: Whole wheat wrap filled with grilled vegetables, chickpeas, and tzatziki sauce

Snack: Roasted edamame beans

Dinner: Turkey meatballs served over zucchini noodles and marinara sauce

Day 4

Breakfast: Spinach and mushroom omelette with whole grain toast

Lunch: Quinoa and black bean salad topped with grilled shrimp

Snack: Homemade trail mix with nuts, dried fruit, and dark chocolate chips

Dinner: Baked tofu served with roasted Brussels sprouts and quinoa

Day 5

Breakfast: Whole grain waffles topped with banana slices and almond butter

Lunch: Vegetable stir-fry with brown rice and cashews

Snack: Cottage cheese with fresh berries

Dinner: Grilled chicken skewers with bell peppers, onions, and pineapple served over a bed of cauliflower rice

Day 6

Breakfast: Spinach and feta omelette with whole grain toast

Lunch: Chickpea and vegetable curry with brown rice

Snack: Banana with peanut butter

Dinner: Baked fish with roasted asparagus and quinoa pilaf

Day 7

Breakfast: Avocado toast on whole grain bread topped with smoked salmon

Lunch: Whole wheat pita filled with hummus, grilled chicken, and vegetables

Snack: Homemade energy balls made with oats, almond butter, and dried fruit

Dinner: Lentil shepherd's pie topped with mashed sweet potatoes.

GLP-1-Friendly Breakfast, Lunch, and Dinner Recipes

Boosting GLP-1 production starts with filling your day with delicious and nutrient-packed meals. Below, you'll find five recipes for breakfast, lunch, and dinner that are simple to prepare, packed with nutrients, and designed to help manage appetite and support hormone health. Each recipe includes ingredients and preparation steps, making it easy to try them out today.

Breakfast Recipes

Avocado & Veggie Scramble

Ingredients:

- 2 eggs (or 3 egg whites)
- ½ small avocado, sliced
- Handful of spinach
- ¼ cup cherry tomatoes, halved
- 1 tsp olive oil
- Salt and pepper to taste

Instructions:

1. Heat olive oil in a pan over medium heat.
2. Add spinach and tomatoes, cooking until softened.
3. Whisk eggs, pour into the pan, and scramble until fully cooked.
4. Serve with avocado slices on top, and season to taste.

Greek Yogurt Parfait with Berries and Walnuts

Ingredients:

- 1 cup of unsweetened Greek yogurt
- ½ cup of a mix of berries like blueberries, raspberries, or strawberries
- 2 tablespoons of finely chopped walnuts
- 1 tablespoon of chia seeds
- Optional drizzle of honey for sweetness

Instructions:

1. Layer yogurt, berries, and walnuts in a bowl or jar.
2. Sprinkle chia seeds on top for an added fiber boost.
3. Drizzle with honey if desired and enjoy.

Overnight Oats with Nut Butter and Banana

Ingredients:

- ½ cup of oatmeal
- ¾ cup of plain almond milk
- 1 small sliced banana
- 1 tablespoon of almond butter or peanut butter
- 1 teaspoon of ground cinnamon

Instructions:

1. Combine oats, almond milk, and cinnamon in a jar or bowl.
2. Top with banana slices and a drizzle of nut butter.
3. Cover and refrigerate overnight. Stir before eating.

High-Protein Green Smoothie

Ingredients:

- 1 cup unsweetened almond milk
- 1 handful of spinach
- ½ avocado
- 1 scoop protein powder (vanilla or unflavored)
- 1 tbsp ground flaxseeds
- ½ cup frozen mango

Instructions:

1. Blend all ingredients until smooth.
2. Pour into a glass and enjoy immediately.

Sweet Potato & Black Bean Breakfast Bowl

Ingredients:

- 1 small sweet potato, peeled and cubed
- ½ cup black beans, cooked
- 1 egg, poached or fried
- 1 tbsp salsa
- 1 tsp olive oil

Instructions:

1. Roast sweet potato cubes with olive oil at 400°F for 20-25 minutes.
2. Add black beans and top with the egg and salsa.
3. Serve warm for a filling breakfast.

Lunch Recipes

Quinoa Kale Salad with Lemon-Tahini Dressing

Ingredients:

- 1 cup cooked quinoa
- 2 cups kale, chopped
- ¼ cup chickpeas
- 2 tbsp tahini
- Juice of ½ lemon
- Salt and pepper to taste

Instructions:

1. Massage kale with a pinch of salt to soften.
2. Combine quinoa, kale, and chickpeas in a bowl.
3. Whisk tahini with lemon juice, adding water to thin if needed, and drizzle over the salad.

Grilled Chicken Lettuce Wraps

Ingredients:

- 1 grilled chicken breast, sliced
- Large butter lettuce leaves
- ½ avocado, diced
- ¼ cup shredded carrots
- Drizzle of salsa or hummus

Instructions:

1. Layer chicken, avocado, and carrots in lettuce leaves.
2. Add a drizzle of salsa or hummus, wrap, and enjoy.

Mediterranean Lentil Bowl

Ingredients:

- 1 cup cooked lentils
- ½ cup cherry tomatoes, halved
- ¼ cucumber, diced
- 1 tbsp olive oil
- 1 tsp balsamic vinegar
- Sprinkle of feta cheese (optional)

Instructions:

1. Combine all ingredients in a bowl and mix well.
2. Top with feta if desired and serve chilled or at room temperature.

Salmon & Sweet Potato Bowl

A filling lunch to keep your energy steady.

Ingredients:

- 1 salmon filet, baked or grilled
- ½ roasted sweet potato, diced
- 1 cup steamed broccoli
- 1 tsp olive oil
- Pinch of salt and pepper

Instructions:

1. Plate the salmon, sweet potato, and broccoli.
2. Drizzle with olive oil, season, and enjoy.

Veggie-Packed Tofu Stir-Fry

Ingredients:

- ½ block firm tofu, cubed
- 1 cup mixed stir-fry vegetables (broccoli, peppers, carrots)
- 1 tbsp soy sauce
- 1 tsp sesame oil
- Sprinkle of sesame seeds

Instructions:

1. Sauté tofu in sesame oil until golden.
2. Add vegetables and stir-fry until tender.
3. Stir in soy sauce, sprinkle with sesame seeds, and serve.

Dinner Recipes

Baked Herb-Crusted Chicken with Veggies

Ingredients:

- 1 chicken breast
- 1 tbsp olive oil
- 1 tsp dried rosemary or thyme
- 1 cup asparagus
- 1 medium baked potato

Instructions:

1. Rub chicken with olive oil and herbs, then bake at 375°F for 25 minutes.
2. Roast asparagus on the side for the last 10 minutes.
3. Serve with a baked potato on the side.

Turkey & Spinach Stuffed Peppers

Ingredients:

- 2 bell peppers, halved and seeded
- 4 oz ground turkey
- 1 cup spinach, chopped
- ½ cup marinara sauce
- ¼ cup shredded mozzarella

Instructions:

1. Cook turkey in a skillet, add spinach, and mix in marinara sauce.
2. Stuff peppers with the mixture, top with mozzarella, and bake at 375°F for 20 minutes.

Pan-Seared Salmon with Quinoa Pilaf

Ingredients:

- 1 salmon filet
- 1 tsp olive oil
- 1 cup cooked quinoa
- ¼ cup chopped parsley
- Juice of ½ lemon

Instructions:

1. Cook salmon in olive oil over medium heat until crispy and flaky.
2. Toss quinoa with parsley and lemon juice, and serve alongside the salmon.

Veggie-Packed Lentil Soup

Ingredients:

- 1 cup lentils, rinsed
- 3 cups vegetable broth
- 1 cup diced carrots
- 1 cup chopped celery
- 1 tsp. cumin

Instructions:

1. Combine all ingredients in a pot and simmer for 30 minutes or until lentils are tender.
2. Serve hot with a side of whole-grain bread if desired.

Zucchini Noodles with Turkey Meatballs

Ingredients:

- 1 zucchini, spiralized
- 4 turkey meatballs (store-bought or homemade)
- ½ cup marinara sauce
- 1 tsp olive oil

Instructions:

1. Heat turkey meatballs in marinara sauce.
2. Sauté spiralized zucchini in olive oil until slightly softened.
3. Serve meatballs and sauce over zucchini noodles.

These recipes are versatile, nutrient-dense, and designed to support GLP-1 activation. Whether you're looking for quick prep or hearty meals, this collection has you covered!

Snack & Drink Ideas That Support Appetite Control

When hunger strikes between meals, the right snack or drink can keep you satisfied while supporting GLP-1 activation. Below, you'll find a variety of options that are nutrient-dense, simple to prepare, and designed to help regulate appetite. These ideas cater to a range of dietary needs and are perfect for busy days when you need something quick and nourishing.

Snack Ideas

Greek Yogurt and Nut Butter Dip with Apple Slices

Ingredients:

- ½ cup plain Greek yogurt
- 1 tbsp almond or peanut butter
- 1 small apple, sliced

Instructions:

1. Mix the yogurt and nut butter in a bowl.
2. Use apple slices as dippers for a creamy, satisfying snack.

Cucumber Boats with Hummus

Ingredients:

- 1 cucumber, halved lengthwise
- 2-3 tbsp hummus

Instructions:

1. Scoop out the seeds of the cucumber halves and fill the "boats" with hummus.
2. Cut into smaller pieces for a grab-and-go option.

Roasted Chickpeas

Ingredients:

- 1 cup canned chickpeas, drained and rinsed
- 1 tbsp olive oil
- 1 tsp paprika or garlic powder

Instructions:

1. Toss chickpeas with olive oil and spices.
2. Roast at 400°F for 25-30 minutes until crispy.

Hard-Boiled Egg and Avocado Slices

Ingredients:

- 1 hard-boiled egg, sliced
- ¼ avocado, sliced
- Pinch of salt and pepper

Instructions:

Arrange egg and avocado slices on a plate, sprinkle with seasoning, and enjoy as a quick and portable snack.

Trail Mix with a Twist

Ingredients:

- ¼ cup raw almonds
- 2 tbsp unsweetened coconut flakes
- 2 tbsp dark chocolate chips

Instructions:

Combine all ingredients in a small bag or container for an on-the-go snack. Opt for portion control to avoid overeating.

Drink Ideas

Protein-Packed Matcha Latte

Ingredients:

- 1 tsp matcha powder
- 1 cup unsweetened almond milk
- 1 scoop of unflavored or vanilla protein powder

Instructions:

Whisk matcha powder with a small amount of hot water, then stir in steamed almond milk and protein powder until smooth.

Fiber-Boosted Green Smoothie

Ingredients:

- 1 cup spinach
- ½ avocado
- 1 cup water or almond milk
- 1 tbsp ground flaxseeds
- Ice cubes

Instructions:

Blend all ingredients until smooth, and enjoy as a nutrient-rich midday sip.

Berry Chia Fresca

Ingredients:

- 2 cups of plain water
- 1 tablespoon of chia seeds
- ½ cup of fresh or frozen berries
- A dash of freshly squeezed lemon juice

Instructions:

Stir chia seeds into water and allow them to soak for 15 minutes before adding berries and lemon. Enjoy chilled.

Golden Almond Milk Latte

Ingredients:

- 1 cup unsweetened almond milk
- ½ tsp turmeric
- ¼ tsp cinnamon
- 1 tsp honey (optional)

Instructions:

1. Heat milk and spices over low heat, whisking until combined.
2. Sweeten with honey if desired and serve warm.

Cucumber Mint Infused Water

Ingredients:

- 1 large pitcher of water
- ½ cucumber, sliced
- 5-6 fresh mint leaves

Instructions:

1. Combine cucumber and mint in water and refrigerate for at least 1 hour before drinking.
2. Great for sipping throughout the day.

Tailoring the Plan for Different Life Stages

Every stage of life brings unique challenges and changes to your body, especially when it comes to weight management, hormones, and metabolism. GLP-1, a hormone that plays a crucial role in appetite control and blood sugar regulation, can be a key player in supporting your health goals. Here, we break down how to optimize GLP-1 activation for women in their 20s and 30s, 40s and 50s, and after menopause.

GLP-1 and Weight Loss in Your 20s & 30s

Your 20s and 30s are often a time of high energy, but balancing work, social life, and personal health can make staying on track challenging. This is also the time when metabolism starts to slow slightly compared to teenage years, so prioritizing healthy habits is key.

How GLP-1 Helps

GLP-1 assists in appetite regulation, helping you feel full after meals. Its role in maintaining stable blood sugar levels also supports consistent energy throughout the day, which is especially important during the busy schedules common in your 20s and 30s.

Strategies to Maximize GLP-1

- *Choose Whole Foods First*: Meals that combine lean protein (like chicken or tofu), healthy fats (avocado, nuts), and complex carbs (quinoa, sweet potatoes) stimulate GLP-1 production and keep you satisfied longer.
- *Stay Active*: Include cardio like running or cycling to keep your metabolism humming, and add strength training to build muscle, which supports GLP-1 activation.
- *Avoid Skipping Meals*: Long gaps between meals can cause blood sugar dips and surges. Aim for balanced meals 3-4 times a day with small snacks in between if needed.
- *Limit Processed Sugars*: Desserts or sugary drinks can interfere with GLP-1's ability to regulate blood sugar effectively, leading to hunger spikes.

Tip for Success

Make meal prepping part of your routine to avoid skipping meals or relying on takeout. Keep quick snacks like trail mix or Greek yogurt handy to curb hunger on busy days.

GLP-1, Hormones, and Metabolism in Your 40s & 50s

During this stage of life, hormonal changes, particularly a decline in estrogen levels, begin to impact metabolism, body composition, and appetite regulation. These changes can make it harder to lose weight and maintain energy levels.

How GLP-1 Helps

GLP-1 plays a key role in counteracting the effects of hormonal fluctuations by balancing appetite and keeping blood sugar levels stable. It also helps prevent overeating, which can become more common during periods of stress or fatigue.

Strategies to Maximize GLP-1

- *Focus on Fiber-Rich Foods*: Fiber supports GLP-1 activation and promotes fullness. Include plenty of vegetables, legumes, and whole grains at every meal.
- *Balance Hormones Naturally*: Incorporate foods rich in phytoestrogens, like soy, flaxseeds, and chickpeas, to help stabilize hormones.
- *Reduce Stress*: Chronic stress raises cortisol levels, which can interfere with GLP-1. Practice relaxation techniques like meditation, yoga, or deep breathing.
- *Be Strategic with Exercise*: Add strength training to preserve muscle mass and combine it with moderate cardio to support heart health and metabolism.

Tip for Success

Create a calming evening routine to support restful sleep. Poor sleep disrupts hunger hormones, making it harder for GLP-1 to do its job effectively. Aim for at least 7-8 hours of quality sleep nightly.

Managing Weight After Menopause

Post-menopause, women experience a marked drop in estrogen levels, which can lead to weight gain, particularly around the abdomen. Additionally, metabolism slows down, making it more challenging to burn calories efficiently.

How GLP-1 Helps

GLP-1 aids in appetite control and can curb overeating, which becomes especially useful when metabolic rates are lower. Its role in blood sugar regulation also helps prevent energy crashes that might otherwise lead to unhealthy snacking.

Strategies to Maximize GLP-1

- *Prioritize Protein*: Protein helps preserve lean muscle mass while stimulating GLP-1. Add options like fish, eggs, beans, and Greek yogurt to your meals.
- *Support Gut Health*: A healthy gut microbiome influences hormone regulation, including GLP-1 production. Include probiotic foods (like yogurt and kimchi) and prebiotic foods (like garlic and oats).

- ***Stay Hydrated***: Proper hydration supports digestion and appetite control. Drink water throughout the day, and try infused waters (like cucumber and mint) for variety.
- ***Adapt Your Portions***: With a slower metabolism, portion sizes may need to be adjusted. Focus on nutrient-dense meals that provide energy without excess calories.

Use smaller plates when serving meals to help with portion control. Fill half your plate with non-starchy vegetables like spinach, broccoli, or zucchini to increase volume without extra calories.

By understanding how GLP-1 functions at different life stages, you can tailor your diet and lifestyle to meet your body's changing needs. Whether you're navigating a fast-paced life in your 20s, addressing hormonal shifts in your 40s, or managing post-menopausal changes, simple adjustments can make a big difference. Focus on nutritious meals, regular activity, and stress management to stay aligned with your health goals.

The Emotional Side of Weight Loss & How to Stay Motivated

Weight loss isn't just about what you eat or how much you exercise. Your emotions, mindset, and motivation play a huge role in shaping the process. For women especially, stress, emotional eating, and unrealistic expectations can create roadblocks that feel hard to overcome. By understanding these challenges and learning how to manage them, you can create a weight-loss experience that feels positive and sustainable.

How Stress and Emotional Eating Affect GLP-1 Levels

Stress and emotional eating are more than just fleeting habits; they can disrupt the hormones that regulate hunger and fullness, including GLP-1. When you're stressed, your body produces higher levels of cortisol, which can interfere with GLP-1's ability to signal satiety. This makes it harder to stop eating, even when your body has had enough.

How Emotional Eating Impacts GLP-1

- ***Temporary Comfort***: Emotional eating is often a quick way to deal with stress, boredom, or sadness. Unfortunately, foods high in sugar and fat provide only temporary relief while potentially dampening GLP-1's ability to regulate your appetite.
- ***Hunger Confusion***: The emotional highs and lows that lead to stress eating can override your body's natural hunger cues, making it hard to know when you're truly hungry or just using food to cope.

Strategies to Break the Cycle

- ***Pause and Reflect***: When the urge to stress eat strikes, take a moment to identify your feelings. Are you truly hungry, or is this an emotional craving? Journaling or talking to a friend can help you process emotions without turning to food.
- ***Choose Balanced Snacks***: If hunger is real, opt for nutrient-dense snacks like Greek yogurt with berries or cucumber slices with hummus, which naturally support GLP-1 production and help you feel satisfied.
- ***Manage Stress Proactively***: Incorporate stress-reducing habits like yoga, deep breathing, or even walking outdoors. These can lower cortisol levels and restore your body's natural rhythm, helping GLP-1 function properly.

The Female Mindset Around Weight Loss: How to Make it Sustainable

For many women, weight loss is tied to deeply ingrained beliefs about body image, self-worth, and societal expectations. These pressures can lead to an all-or-nothing mindset that makes setbacks feel like failures.

Building a Positive and Sustainable Mindset

- *Shift the Focus to Health*: Instead of focusing solely on numbers (weight, calories), think about how you feel in your body. Are your meals giving you energy? Do your workouts make you feel strong? These achievements matter more than a number on the scale.
- *Reframe Setbacks*: Instead of viewing a missed workout or indulgent meal as a failure, see it as part of the process. Progress comes from consistency, not perfection.
- *Find Joy in Movement*: Weight loss doesn't have to mean punishing workouts. Choose activities you genuinely enjoy, like dancing, hiking, or swimming. When fitness feels fun, it's easier to stick with it.
- *Celebrate Non-Scale Victories*: Notice and celebrate changes beyond weight, like better sleep, improved mood, or reduced stress levels. These victories are often the first signs of lasting health improvements.

Realistic Expectations and Avoiding Burnout

Starting a weight-loss journey often comes with high hopes and ambitious goals. But when progress feels slow or doesn't match your expectations, it's easy to get discouraged. Setting realistic goals is critical to avoid burnout and stay motivated for the long haul. Remember, lasting health is a marathon, not a sprint.

Why Unrealistic Expectations Can Lead to Burnout

- *Comparison Traps on Social Media*: Scrolling through photos of dramatic transformations can make your progress feel inadequate. But remember, those posts often don't show the full story. Real health improvements happen gradually, at a pace unique to your body, and that's okay.
- *Unsustainable Routines*: Crash diets and extreme workouts might yield quick results, but they're tough to maintain. Pushing yourself too hard can lead to physical and mental exhaustion, making it even harder to stay on track.

Unrealistic goals can overshadow the small victories that truly matter on your health journey. By shifting your perspective, you can avoid burnout and create a plan you enjoy sticking with.

How to Set Realistic Expectations

1. ***Focus on Progress, Not Perfection***: Health is built on small, consistent changes. Celebrate progress like losing 1–2 pounds per week, cooking balanced meals regularly, or moving your body more frequently. These steps add up and create a foundation for long-term success.
2. ***Prioritize Balance Over Extremes***: Sustainability is key. You don't have to give up your favorite foods or punish yourself for indulging. Instead, aim for balanced eating that includes room for enjoyment. Cravings and flexibility are part of a healthy lifestyle.
3. ***Track How You Feel, Not Just Numbers***: The scale doesn't tell the whole story. Use a journal to note improvements in mood, energy levels, sleep quality, or even confidence. These "non-scale victories" are often the first signs that your efforts are paying off.

Recognizing Signs of Burnout

It's normal to feel a little worn out sometimes, but if any of these signs persist, it might be time to hit pause and reassess your routine:

- Feeling constantly tired or unmotivated
- Losing interest in the activities you once enjoyed
- Criticizing yourself harshly for small setbacks

Taking care of yourself also means recognizing when you need to rest—not push harder.

How to Reset and Recharge

If burnout starts creeping in, shift gears. It's not about giving up; it's about finding balance. Here's how to move forward without losing your momentum:

- *Adjust Your Routine*: If workouts feel draining, switch to something gentler like yoga or walking. If strict meal plans are overwhelming, simplify your meals or try meal prep to lighten the load.
- *Schedule Rest Days*: Rest isn't a weakness; it's a form of self-care. Build breaks into your schedule so your body and mind can recover.
- *Seek Support*: A loved one, friend, or coach can help you regroup and refocus. Sometimes, an encouraging voice is all you need to stay grounded.

Focusing on the emotional side of weight loss is essential for building habits that last. Find tools and strategies that work for you, lean on supportive people in your life, and treat yourself with care. Motivation isn't about staying driven every single day; it's about remembering why you started and finding ways to reconnect to your goals when life gets overwhelming.

Troubleshooting Common Challenges

Navigating a health or weight-loss plan is rarely a straight path. Challenges are a natural part of the process, and understanding how to manage them can make all the difference. Here's a closer look at some common obstacles, along with practical strategies to help you stay on track.

Not Seeing Results? Adjustments for Your Body

It can be frustrating when your progress slows or stalls, even when you're sticking to your plan. Weight loss isn't always linear, and plateaus are often a sign that your body is adapting to changes. A few thoughtful adjustments may help get things moving again.

Why Progress Slows

- *Unnoticed Calorie Creep*: Portion sizes or hidden calories in sauces, dressings, and snacks can add up quickly.

- *Metabolic Adaptations*: Over time, your body may adjust to a lower calorie intake, making it harder to see changes.
- *Routine Stagnation*: Sticking to the same workouts or meal plans can lead to reduced effectiveness.

Strategies to Reignite Progress

- *Evaluate Portions*: Take a closer look at portion sizes or log meals for a few days to ensure you're on track. Be mindful of calorie-dense foods like nuts and oils.
- *Diversify Your Exercise*: If your routine has become predictable, try mixing in new activities. Switching between strength training, cardio, or high-intensity workouts can challenge your body in fresh ways.
- *Introduce Variety to Meals*: Experiment with different proteins, vegetables, and whole grains to keep your nutrition diverse and prevent nutrient gaps.
- *Prioritize Sleep and Stress Management*: Rest and recovery are just as critical as diet and exercise. Lack of sleep or high stress can disrupt hormones, impacting your progress.

Even small adjustments can yield significant results. Trust the process and keep experimenting to find what works for your body.

How to Overcome Hunger, Fatigue, or Energy Dips

Feeling hungry, tired, or drained can be discouraging, but it doesn't mean your plan isn't working. These sensations are often signals from your body that adjustments are needed to support energy balance and appetite regulation.

Managing Persistent Hunger

- *Boost Protein Intake*: Protein helps you stay fuller for longer. Include a source at every meal, such as eggs, chicken, tofu, or beans.
- *Increase Fiber*: Foods like lentils, chia seeds, leafy greens, and whole grains can promote satiety and regulate blood sugar.
- *Stay Hydrated*: Sometimes thirst is mistaken for hunger. Drinking water before meals can help curb cravings.
- *Balance Your Plate*: A combination of protein, healthy fats, fiber, and complex carbs provides steady energy and keeps hunger at bay.

Addressing Fatigue and Energy Dips

- *Avoid Refined Carbs*: Foods like white bread or sugary snacks may provide a quick energy boost, but they often lead to crashes. Opt for slow-digesting options like oats, nuts, or yogurt instead.

- *Eat Regularly*: Spacing meals 3–4 hours apart can stabilize blood sugar and prevent sluggishness.
- *Check for Nutrient Deficiencies*: Fatigue can result from low levels of iron or B vitamins. Include iron-rich foods like spinach or supplemented cereal, along with foods like eggs or fish for B vitamins.
- *Move More*: A brisk walk, even for 10 minutes, can counteract energy dips after a meal, especially lunch.

Paying attention to hunger cues and energy levels allows you to make smarter adjustments that still fit within your goals.

Signs Your GLP-1 Activation Needs Extra Support

GLP-1 (glucagon-like peptide-1) plays a vital role in controlling hunger, stabilizing blood sugar, and supporting weight management. However, some signs may suggest that your body needs help bolstering GLP-1 activity.

Indicators of Poor GLP-1 Activation

- *Constant Hunger*: If hunger returns soon after meals despite balanced portions, GLP-1 signaling may need support.
- *Uncontrolled Cravings*: Intense cravings for sugar or fatty foods could mean hunger regulation is off.

- ***Energy Crashes***: Sudden dips in energy between meals may suggest GLP-1 isn't stabilizing blood sugar levels effectively.
- ***Plateaued Weight Loss***: When no significant progress occurs despite maintaining your plan, GLP-1 could be influenced by other factors like stress or diet quality.

Supporting Healthy GLP-1 Activation

- ***Opt for Smaller, Frequent Meals***: Consuming smaller, well-balanced meals throughout the day can encourage steadier GLP-1 hormone levels.
- ***Focus on Gut Health***: Foods rich in probiotics, like yogurt, kefir, and kimchi, can improve gut microbial activity, which interacts with GLP-1 production.
- ***Stay Active***: Exercise boosts GLP-1 activity, so aim to incorporate regular workouts, including strength training and cardio.
- ***Avoid Highly Processed Foods***: Stick to natural and whole ingredients, as refined products can interfere with GLP-1 responses.
- ***Include Healthy Fats***: Avocados, nuts, olive oil, and seeds support metabolic function and encourage satiety.

When to Seek Extra Guidance

If consistent efforts don't seem to help, or if symptoms like fatigue or persistent hunger continue, consulting with a healthcare provider or nutrition expert may identify if there are underlying conditions like insulin resistance or hormonal imbalances that need addressing.

Challenges are part of any meaningful change, but they're not insurmountable. With the right adjustments and a willingness to adapt, you can continue progressing towards your goals. Listen to your body's signals, don't hesitate to troubleshoot, and remember that setbacks are just opportunities to learn what works best for you.

Beyond 30 Days – Making the GLP-1 Lifestyle Sustainable

The first 30 days of any health or weight-loss program often focus on learning the ropes, building momentum, and seeing early results. But the real magic happens when you transform short-term changes into a sustainable way of life. This chapter dives into how to make the GLP-1 lifestyle part of your long-term routine, create lasting healthy habits, and harness natural strategies to support women's health.

Transitioning from a Short-Term Plan to a Lifelong Strategy

While structured plans can be helpful at the start, long-term success depends on moving beyond rigid methods and adapting behaviors to fit into your everyday life. Here's how to make the shift:

1. **Focus on Consistency, Not Perfection**

    Life is unpredictable, and no one eats perfectly or exercises without fail every day. Rather than aiming for perfection, focus on consistency. Make small, manageable choices most of the time, like choosing a nutrient-dense meal or going for a quick walk, even on busy days.

2. **Adjust and Adapt Over Time**

   Your needs may evolve as your body, goals, and circumstances change. View this process as flexible and fluid. For example, you might need to tweak your meal plans, try different forms of exercise, or reevaluate your calorie and macronutrient needs down the road.

3. **Make Enjoyment a Priority**

   Your health routine should feel rewarding, not like a chore. Find foods you love that align with your plan, and experiment with exercises that bring you joy, whether that's dancing, hiking, or strength training. The more you enjoy the process, the more likely you are to stick with it.

4. **Celebrate Progress in All Forms**

   Remember, success isn't measured by the scale alone. Celebrate the non-scale victories like improved energy, better sleep, reduced stress, or a boost in confidence. These wins are just as important and will keep you motivated as you build a sustainable lifestyle.

Building a lifelong strategy is about staying flexible, consistent, and finding joy in the process. Focus on small, sustainable changes and celebrate every step forward, no matter how big or small.

Building Healthy Habits That Last

Forming habits is less about willpower and more about creating systems that work for you. When these habits become second nature, you can support your health goals with less effort and stress.

1. **Start Small and Build Gradually**

    Big overhauls are hard to sustain. Instead, focus on one change at a time. For instance, start by adding a serving of vegetables to lunch, then work on drinking more water the next week. Over time, small steps add up to significant, lasting change.

2. **Lean on Routine**

    Routine makes healthy habits easier to maintain. Try setting specific times for meals, workouts, or self-care activities. For example, make morning walks part of your day or prepare healthy lunches on Sundays. Predictable routines reduce decision fatigue and help you stay consistent.

3. **Create an Environment for Success**

    Your surroundings can support or sabotage your goals. Keep healthy snacks within reach, stock your kitchen with nutritious options, and remove tempting foods that don't align with your objectives. Create spaces that encourage movement, like leaving a yoga mat visible as a reminder to stretch or exercise.

4. **Be Patient and Forgiving**

    Habits take time to solidify. Research shows it can take weeks or even months before a new behavior feels automatic. If you slip up, don't dwell on it. Focus on getting back on track with your next choice. Remember, it's the overall pattern of your behavior that matters most, not one-off setbacks.

Building healthy habits takes time, patience, and small, consistent steps. Focus on creating systems and environments that support your goals, and remember that progress is about persistence, not perfection.

Other Natural Hormone Hacks for Women's Health

The GLP-1 pathway is just one piece of the puzzle when it comes to hormonal health. A few additional strategies can support overall wellness and make it easier to maintain weight management long term.

1. **Prioritize Gut Health**

   Your gut and hormones are closely connected, influencing everything from GLP-1 production to mood regulation. Boost gut health by eating plenty of fiber, fermented foods (like yogurt or sauerkraut), and prebiotics (such as bananas and asparagus). Reducing processed foods and added sugars can also support a healthy gut microbiome.

2. **Balance Your Blood Sugar**

   Keeping blood sugar levels steady helps regulate energy and metabolism. Maintain balance by pairing carbs with protein and healthy fats, which slow digestion and prevent spikes. For example, combine an apple with nut butter or pair whole-grain toast with eggs.

3. **Manage Stress Levels**

   Chronic stress increases cortisol, which can interfere with hormones like insulin and GLP-1. Incorporate stress-reducing practices such as mindfulness, yoga, or even short breathing exercises throughout your day. Find what helps you feel calm and relaxed.

4. **Support Sleep Quality**

   Sleep is essential for hormone balance and overall health. Poor sleep can impact hunger hormones like ghrelin, leading to increased cravings. Set a regular sleep schedule, limit screen time before bed, and create a calming bedtime routine to improve rest.

5. **Include Hormone-Friendly Foods**

   Certain nutrients play a key role in hormone health. Foods rich in omega-3 fatty acids (like salmon or flaxseeds), magnesium (in spinach and nuts), and vitamin D (from fortified foods or sunlight) can support hormonal functions and overall wellness.

Sustainability is the foundation of a healthy lifestyle, and making small, realistic changes over time is the best way to maintain progress. By transitioning from a short-term focus to a lifelong strategy, building habits that align with your goals, and incorporating natural ways to support your hormones, you can create a lifestyle that not only works for you but that you genuinely enjoy.

Remember, this is your unique health journey. Go at your own pace, listen to your body, and trust that consistency and care will yield lasting results.

Conclusion

Thank you for reading through this guide and exploring how GLP-1 can support your health and wellness goals. By taking the time to understand this hormone's role in appetite regulation, energy levels, and weight management, you've equipped yourself with practical strategies that align with your body's needs. You've also gained insight into the unique challenges women face, from hormonal fluctuations to societal expectations, and how to approach them with tailored solutions.

The most important takeaway is that your health is a personal and evolving process. What works for someone else might not fully suit you, and that's okay. The key is experimenting, listening to your body, and implementing small, sustainable changes over time. Whether it's adjusting your diet, incorporating more movement into your day, or simply prioritizing sleep and stress management, incremental steps create impactful, lasting progress. There's no need to rush or strive for perfection. Instead, focus on building habits that feel natural and manageable for you.

It's also crucial to remember that progress isn't measured solely by weight loss. Celebrate changes like better energy levels, improved mood, fewer cravings, or feeling stronger during your workouts. These victories may seem subtle, but they're powerful indicators that your efforts are making a genuine difference. Health is a holistic pursuit, and these milestones reinforce how interconnected physical and emotional well-being truly are.

As you continue on this path, stay flexible and open-minded. Every stage of life brings new demands, whether it's busy days in your 20s and 30s, hormonal shifts in your 40s and 50s, or the physical changes that come post-menopause. The good news is that with the knowledge you've gained here, you're better prepared to adapt your habits to fit your current needs. Whether you're tweaking your meal plan or rethinking your exercise routine, small adjustments can keep you aligned with your goals.

Along the way, give yourself room for setbacks. They're not failures but opportunities to learn and refine your approach. It's natural for motivation to waver, and progress may not always be linear—but what matters is persistence and the decision to keep putting in the effort. The focus shouldn't be on temporary fixes, but on creating a sustainable way of living that supports your overall health, emotionally and physically.

If this guide has given you clarity and practical tools, use them as a starting point. Keep building on what works for you while remaining curious and adaptable. Change is a process, and every thoughtful choice you make brings you closer to the health and balance you aim for.

Thank you for allowing this guide to be part of your wellness efforts. Continue to seek progress over perfection, prioritize what makes sense for you, and celebrate how far you've come. Every positive step counts, and with the resilience and knowledge you've developed, you're more than capable of achieving a sustainable and fulfilling lifestyle. Keep moving forward—you're well on your way.

FAQs

What is GLP-1, and why is it important for weight management?

GLP-1, or glucagon-like peptide-1, is a natural hormone produced in your gut. It helps regulate appetite, blood sugar, and energy balance by communicating with your brain to signal fullness and stabilizing glucose levels. Understanding GLP-1 allows you to leverage its effects to manage cravings and support sustainable weight loss.

Can the GLP-1 diet work for all women, regardless of age?

Yes, the GLP-1 diet is adaptable to different life stages. Women in their 20s, 30s, 40s, and post-menopause can tailor the diet to meet their changing needs by focusing on hormone-friendly foods, meal timing, and exercise. The personalized approach ensures it supports wherever you are in your health journey.

What types of foods are considered GLP-1-friendly?

Foods high in fiber, healthy fats, lean proteins, and probiotics are excellent for boosting GLP-1 production. Examples include vegetables, fruits, whole grains, fatty fish, nuts, seeds, Greek yogurt, and fermented foods like kimchi or sauerkraut. These foods enhance appetite control and promote gut health.

How can I naturally activate GLP-1 without medications?

You can boost GLP-1 levels by eating balanced, nutrient-dense meals, staying physically active, managing stress, and getting enough sleep. Simple habits like spacing meals evenly, drinking plenty of water, and including fiber and protein in your diet can naturally enhance GLP-1 secretion.

Will I still lose weight if I don't follow the meal plan exactly?

Yes! The GLP-1 diet isn't about strict rules but rather creating a sustainable approach that works for you. Small, consistent improvements, such as incorporating GLP-1-friendly foods or adjusting meal timing, can lead to steady progress. Customize the plan to align with your lifestyle and preferences.

Is fasting necessary to follow the GLP-1 diet successfully?

Fasting isn't required but can be helpful for some women. Techniques like intermittent fasting (e.g., 12/12 or 16/8) can give your body time to optimize GLP-1 production, manage blood sugar levels, and control hunger. It's entirely optional and should only be practiced if it feels natural for you.

How long before I see results with the GLP-1 diet?

Results vary depending on your body, consistency, and other factors like exercise and stress levels. Many women experience better appetite control, fewer cravings, or improved energy within a few weeks. Sustainable weight loss typically happens gradually, with visible changes often occurring after the first month.

References and Helpful Links

Professional, C. C. M. (2025b, March 19). GLP-1 agonists. Cleveland Clinic. https://my.clevelandclinic.org/health/treatments/13901-glp-1-agonists

Do men really lose weight more easily than women? (n.d.). https://www.texashealth.org/Health-and-Wellness/Bariatrics/Do-Men-Really-Lose-Weight-More-Easily-Than-Women

Pedersen, T. (2024, March 13). What foods increase GLP-1 levels? Healthline. https://www.healthline.com/health/foods-that-increase-glp-1

Xie, Y., Choi, T., & Al-Aly, Z. (2025). Mapping the effectiveness and risks of GLP-1 receptor agonists. Nature Medicine. https://doi.org/10.1038/s41591-024-03412-w

Courtney. (2025, January 31). Study identifies benefits, risks linked to popular weight-loss drugs | WashU Medicine. WashU Medicine. https://medicine.washu.edu/news/study-identifies-benefits-risks-linked-to-popular-weight-loss-drugs/

Mills, D. (2025, January 21). GLP-1 drugs benefit brain and heart health, but may cause kidney, GI issues. Healthline. https://www.healthline.com/health-news/glp-1-drugs-benefits-risks-health-outcomes

News-Medical. (2025, March 19). The unexpected effects of GLP-1 medications on women's health. https://www.news-medical.net/health/The-Unexpected-Effects-of-GLP-1-Medications-on-Womene28099s-Health.aspx

Achieve and maintain your weight loss goals with GLP-1 medications: women's health specialists, PLLC: OBGYNs. (n.d.). https://www.whstn.com/blog/achieve-and-maintain-your-weight-loss-goals-with-glp-1-medications

Rd, E. L. M. (2025, February 27). Simple 7-Day GLP-1-Friendly meal plan for beginners, created by a dietitian. EatingWell. https://www.eatingwell.com/simple-7-day-glp-1-friendly-meal-plan-for-beginners-11681814

www.ingramcontent.com/pod-product-compliance
Lightning Source LLC
LaVergne TN
LVHW012029060526
838201LV00061B/4522